Gastroenterology:
Fast Focus Study Guide

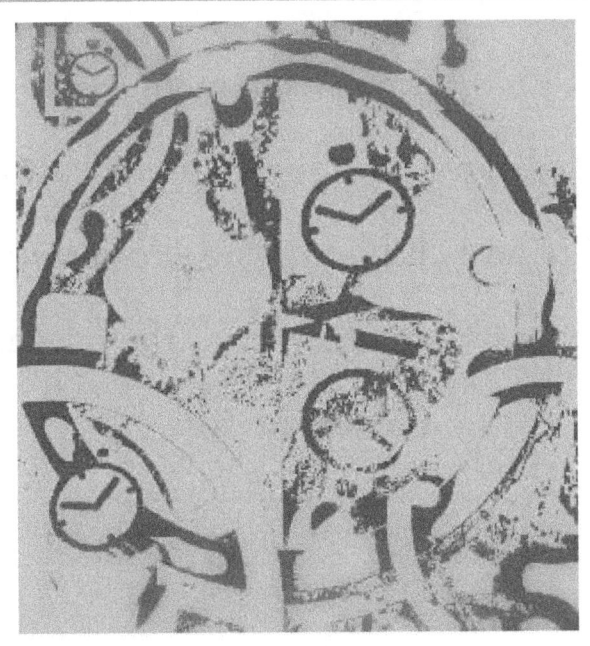

Acknowledgements

I dedicate this book to my beautiful
wife and children, who I love more
than all the water in all the oceans
and all the seas.

CONTENTS

- This book is written for any medical professionals who want to learn more about Gastroenterology.

- There are over 300 pages of easy to read facts about Gastroenterology.

- Put this book in your bathroom or on your coffee table.

- This is the perfect graduation gift for the aspiring physician or graduating physician.

- This Fast Focus Study Guide will provide you with a practical review of the key information you need to know.

- Buy this book now if you want this quick and concise information

What is the motility disorder of the esophagus associated with impaired relaxation of the lower esophageal sphincter?

Achalasia

What is the underlying pathophysiology of achalasia?

Loss of innervation to the lower esophageal sphincter (Auerbach's plexus is lost) and failure of relaxation of Auerbach's plexus

What are the radiographic findings of achalasia?

Achalasia is associated with birds beak narrowing at the gastroesophageal junction on a barium swallow

How can you tell small bowel from large bowel on abdominal x-ray?

Small bowel plicae conniventes are complete. Large bowel plicae semilunares are only partially around the inner circumference of the lumen

What are sentinel loops on an abdominal radiograph?

Distension and/or air-fluid levels in bowel near a site of abdominal inflammation

What is the obturator sign?

The obturator sign is described as pain upon internal rotation of leg with hip and knee flexed. It is associated with peritonitis and is commonly seen in the setting of appendicitis and pelvic abscess.

Which disorder is characterized by post prandial RUQ pain, bilious vomiting, anemia, steatorrhea, and pain which resolves suddenly after decompression?

Afferent loop syndrome (common after billroth II)

How does viral hepatitis affect the AST: ALT ratio?

Viral hepatitis will generally result in an equal increase in both ALT and AST resulting in an AST: ALT ratio of 0.5-0.8

How is the ALT affected by pyridoxine (B6) deficiency?

Pyridoxine deficiency can result in a decrease in the ALT levels

How often is the ALT increased in patients receiving heparin?

Approximately 60% of these patients will have a mild increase in their ALT

Is the ALT a more specific indicator of liver damage than the AST?

Yes

What conditions should be considered when the AST is elevated more than the ALT?

Non hepatic etiology such as celiac sprue, acquired muscle diseases, and recent strenuous exercises should be considered in the differential diagnosis

What happens to the ALT in response to hepatocellular injury?

Hepatocellular injury results in a rise in the ALT

What is the most common etiology
when the AST: ALT ratio is between
2 and 6?

Alcoholic liver disease

Which antibiotics are associated with rises in the ALT and AST?

Ketoconazole, fluconazole, isoniazid, synthetic penicillin, ciprofloxacin, and nitrofurantoin can result in an increase in the hepatic enzymes

Which anticonvulsant drugs are associated with rises in the ALT and AST?

Phenytoin and carbamazepine can result in increases in the hepatic enzymes

What is the half-life of albumin?

The half-life of albumin is 15-19 days

Which 3 causes of cirrhosis are associated with long and detailed family histories of liver disease?

-Hemochromatosis

-Alpha 1 antitrypsin deficiency

-Wilson's disease

Does the blood for ammonia measurement need special handling?

Yes, it should be placed on ice immediately after drawing

How is ammonia normally metabolized in the body?

Ammonia is normally transported from the colon to the liver where hepatocytes metabolize it to urea

What are some causes of increased blood ammonia?

Increased blood ammonia can most commonly result from decreased destruction of ammonia (liver disease) or by increased production of ammonia (GI bleed)

Where is ammonia normally produced in the body?

Ammonia is normally produced by bacteria in the colon

What condition is defined by the pancreas encircling the duodenum?

Annular pancreas

How often do adults develop appendiceal perforation related to an appendicitis?

Approximately 20% of adults with an appendicitis will develop appendiceal perforation

How often will patients with an appendicitis initially present with periumbilical pain?

Approximately 50% of patients will initially have periumbilical pain

What is the most common surgical emergency?

Appendicitis

What is the psoas sign which can be
positive in patients with appendicitis?

Pain with right thigh extension

What is the Rovsing's sign which can be positive in patients with appendicitis?

The Rovsing's sign is pain in the right lower quadrant with palpation in the left lower quadrant

What percentage of patients develop appendicitis because of a foreign body such as a pin worm or fruit seed obstructing the appendiceal lumen?

Approximately 4% of patients have appendicitis related to a foreign body

What percentage of patients develop appendicitis because of fecalith obstruction the appendiceal lumen?

Approximately 30-35% of appendicitis are related to fecaliths

What percentage of the population will develop appendicitis?

Approximately 10% of the population

What are irregularly shaped clusters of arterial, venous, and capillary vessels within the submucosa of bowel wall which most often occur in the right colon of elderly Caucasian patients?

Colonic arteriovenous malformation

What are three types of ascites?

Exudative ascites

Transudative ascites

Chylous ascites

List five causes of transudative ascites?

Cirrhosis; Chronic hepatic congestion (Budd-Chiari, constrictive pericarditis, right heart failure); Nephrotic syndrome; Myxedema; Meigs syndrome

List four causes of exudative ascites?

TB peritonitis; Pancreatitis; Ruptured viscera; Tumors (most commonly metastatic to liver and peritoneal cavity)

What are two causes of chylous ascites?

-Trauma of the thoracic duct or abdominal lymphatics

-Mediastinal tumors

What are two conditions that commonly cause pancreatic ascites?

Leaking pseudocyst; Tear in pancreatic duct

What are two parameters diagnostic
of pancreatic ascites?

Ascitic fluid amylase >1000;
Sometimes normal serum amylase

What is the probable etiology of
ascites in a patient with a history of
alcohol abuse presenting with new
onset ascites, stable liver function
tests, and no hepatomegaly?

Pancreatic ascites

What can lessen the potential for aspiration in a patient receiving nasogastric tube feedings?

Placing the tube in the duodenum

Which disorder is characterized by destruction of the squamous epithelium of the distal esophagus which is replaced with columnar epithelium? Adenocarcinoma may develop in 2-5% of these patients?

Barrett's esophagus

Blind loop syndrome is attributed to overgrowth of bacteria in the small intestine. What are five characteristic findings?

Malabsorption of B12; Steatorrhea; Hypoproteinemia; Weight loss; Diarrhea

What is Boerhaave's syndrome?

Boerhaave's syndrome is characterized by rupture of the distal esophagus in a patient who has had forceful retching

What is the most common location of Boerhaave's syndrome?

Posterior-lateral aspect of esophagus on left 3-5 cm above the GE junction

Which disease is associated with occlusion of the IVC or hepatic veins, leading to congestive liver disease with necrosis around the central vein?

Budd-Chiari syndrome

List six agents that cause diarrhea by activating the adenylate cyclase/CAMP system?

Cholera toxin; E. coli heat labile toxin; Vasoactive intestinal polypeptide; Prostaglandins; Salmonella enterotoxin; Dihydroxy bile acids and fatty acids

List two methods by which cyclic-AMP produces secretory diarrhea?

CAMP can inhibit absorption of fluids from the GI tract and/or stimulate secretion of sodium and chloride

What is the most common infection of the esophagus?

Candida albicans

What is a caput medusae?

A caput medusae is characterized by congestion and engorgement of the superficial periumbilical vein associated with portal hypertension caused by liver failure

IgA and IgG anti-gliadin antibodies are increased in more than 90% of patients, but are not specific. What is a better blood test for celiac disease?

IgA endomysial antibodies are the best screening blood test to diagnose celiac disease

Is there an increased risk of lymphoma in patients with celiac disease?

Yes, these patients are at increased risk for small bowel T-cell lymphoma

What disorder is characterized by gliadin sensitivity associated with destruction of surface intestinal epithelial cells, blunted and flat villi, and crypt hypertrophy?

Celiac disease (diagnosis requires 3 sequential small intestine biopsies showing flattened mucosa abdominal recovery of mucosa after gluten free diet for 12 months)

What are the components of
Charcot's triad for cholangitis?

- Fever/chills

- Jaundice

- RUQ pain

What is cholangitis?

Cholangitis is a bacterial infection of the biliary tract that usually occurs in the setting of obstructed ducts

What is the most common bacterial etiology of cholangitis?

E. coli is the most common cause of cholangitis; 1/4 are caused by anaerobes, the most common of which is Bacillus fragilis

What is the most common cause of
common bile duct obstruction?

Gall stones

Murphy's sign is pain in RUQ during inspiration, while palpating under right costal margin. What clinical condition is it often seen with?

Acute cholecystitis

What disorder is associated with acute cholecystitis without evidence of stones, believed to be secondary to sludge in the gallbladder?

Acalculous cholecystitis

What is acalculous cholecystitis?

Acalculous cholecystitis is characterized by inflammation of the gallbladder without gall stones

What is the definition of cholecystitis?

Cholecystitis is inflammation of the gallbladder

What is the most common cause of acute cholecystitis?

Acute cholecystitis is most commonly due to cystic duct obstruction secondary to an impacted gallstone

What is the definition of choledocholithiasis?

Choledocholithiasis is defined as presence of gall stones in the common bile duct

What are the most common type of gall stones?

Cholesterol gall stones account for 75% of gall stones. These stones occur secondary to bile that is super saturated with cholesterol. Cholesterol stones are radiolucent.

Which type of small bowel obstruction can occur when a large gallstone erodes through the gallbladder and into the duodenum/small bowel?

Gall stone Ileus

How often do patients with chronic active hepatitis from autoimmune etiology have an anti-smooth muscle antibody?

Approximately 50-80% of patients with chronic active hepatitis have anti smooth muscle antibody

How often do patients with viral hepatitis have anti smooth-muscle antibody?

Only 1:25 of patients with viral hepatitis have anti-smooth muscle antibodies

Describe chronic pancreatitis?

Inflammation of the pancreas secondary to auto digestion by its own activated enzymes causing destruction of parenchyma with fibrosis and calcification leading to an eventual decrease in endocrine and exocrine function

Hepatic failure may lead to these secondary conditions?

Hyperammonemia; Hepatic encephalopathy; Hypoglycemia; Impaired absorption of long chain fatty acids

In liver disease, what causes a decrease in red cells, white cells, and platelets?

Splenic sequestration

In liver disease, what causes spider telangiectasias and palmar erythema?

Altered estrogen and androgen metabolism with altered vascular physiology

List 8 causes of cirrhosis?

ETOH; Hepatic viruses; Drugs;
Autoimmune chronic active hepatitis;
Biliary cirrhosis; Chronic hepatic
congestion; Genetically determined
metabolic disease; Cryptogenic

List five common vitamins that are often deficient in the setting of liver disease?

Folic acid; Vitamin B6; Thiamine; Sometimes Vitamin D; Zinc

List four genetic diseases known to cause cirrhosis?

Hemochromatosis; Wilson's disease; alpha 1-antitrypsin deficiency; galactosemia

What are three causes of chronic hepatic congestion that are known to cause cirrhosis?

Budd Chiari syndrome; chronic right heart failure; Constrictive pericarditis

What causes gynecomastia, testicular atrophy, and decreased libido in liver disease?

Altered estrogen and androgen metabolism.

What causes hypoglycemia in patients
with underlying liver disease?

Decreased glycogen stores and
decreased gluconeogenesis

What in the most common cause of GI bleeding among patients with underlying liver disease?

Esophageal varices

What is a common cause of
ecchymosis in the setting of liver
disease?

Decreased synthesis of clotting factors

What is the classical difference
between the causes of micronodular
cirrhosis and macronodular cirrhosis?

Micronodular cirrhosis occurs in the
setting of chronic insult (ETOH).
Macronodular cirrhosis is usually
caused by an acute insult.

What are the two types of biliary cirrhosis?

Primary biliary cirrhosis; Secondary biliary cirrhosis (bile duct strictures, sclerosing cholangitis, biliary atresia, tumors of bile ducts,) cystic fibrosis

What are the three types of benign adenomatous polyps seen on colonoscopy?

-Tubular adenoma (75%)

-Tubulovillous (15%)

-Villous adenoma (10%)

What are three preventative and early detection procedures for the detection of colorectal cancer?

Annual digital rectal exam starting at age 40; Occult blood testing at age 40; Sigmoidoscopy or colonoscopy at 50, then every 3-5 years

What is the most common cause of colonic (large bowel) obstruction in adults?

Colorectal cancer

Where is the pain from rectal disease often referred?

Rectal pain is often referred to the small of the back

What are the signs and symptoms of intestinal obstruction?

Intestinal obstruction is often associated with vomiting, obstipation, distention, cramping, and abdominal pain

What are the three most common causes of colonic obstruction?

Sigmoid diverticulitis; Sigmoid volvulus; Colon carcinoma

What is the definition of constipation?

Constipation is less than 3 bowel movements per week

Which classes of drugs are most commonly associated with constipation?

Iron supplements, antacids, and calcium channel blockers are commonly associated. Anticholinergic medications such as cold remedies, antidepressants, opioids and antipsychotics are also associated with constipation.

Which disorder is due to absent UDP glucuronyl transferase resulting in an unconjugated hyperbilirubinemia?

Crigler-Najjar syndrome

How often do patients with Crohn's disease and ulcerative colitis develop peripheral arthritis?

Approximately 20% of patients with Crohn's disease and ulcerative colitis will develop associated peripheral arthritis

List three GI manifestations of Diabetes?

Disturbances of esophageal motility; Gastroparesis with delayed gastric emptying; Diarrhea (usually nocturnal)

Describe three pathogenic
mechanisms of bacteria/parasitic
diarrhea?

Toxins; Adherence to intestinal
mucosa; Invasion

Name two mechanisms that will decrease absorptive surface in the GI and possibly cause inadequate absorption?

Bowel resection; enteric fistula

Stool osmotic gap suggests an osmotic cause of diarrhea due to short chain fatty acids or carbohydrates. How do you calculate the stool osmotic gap?

Plasma Osmolarity - 2 (stool Na + K) = Stool Osmolarity

What are five organisms that invade mucosa and result in diarrhea?

Salmonella; Shigella; Enteropathic E. coli; Campylobacter; Yersinia

What is the most common cause of Campylobacter enteritis?

Campylobacter jejuni is the most common cause of Campylobacter enteritis.

What cause of diarrhea is due to destruction of the mucosa, with impaired absorption, and outpouring of blood and mucous? It is associated with fever and small frequent stools with blood and pus?

Inflammatory diarrhea is associated with these symptoms and can be caused by ulcerative colitis, shigellosis, or amebiasis

What condition is associated with diarrhea and buccal pigmentation?

Peutz-Jegher's syndrome

What disorder is characterized by non-absorbable molecules in the gut lumen, watery stool without blood or pus? This diarrhea improves with fasting and the stool may contain fat globules or meat fibers and may have an increased solute gap?

Osmotic diarrhea (lactose intolerance, generalized malabsorption, magnesium containing laxatives)

What is the most common cause of traveler's diarrhea?

Enterotoxigenic E. Coli is the most common cause of traveler's diarrhea.

What is the most common cause of

infectious diarrhea in the US?

Campylobacter jejuni

What type of diarrhea is suggested by resolution of diarrhea after a 2-3 day fast?

Osmotic diarrhea should be considered in this setting

When fecal white cells are noted on exam, what are two possible causes?

-Infection

-Inflammatory bowel disease

Which type of diarrhea is associated with increased motility and decreased time for absorption of electrolytes and/or nutrients? It is also associated with decreased motility with bacterial overgrowth resulting in malabsorption?

Dysmotility diarrhea (hyperthyroidism, irritable bowel syndrome, scleroderma, diabetic diarrhea)

Define the diverticula of the colon?

These are present in 50-60% of people by the age of 60. The diverticula of the colon are false diverticula because only the mucosa and submucosa herniate through the bowel wall.

These occur secondary to weakness where the blood vessels enter between antimesenteric and mesenteric tenia.

What disorder is characterized by herniation of colonic mucosa and submucosa through muscularis, generally found along the colon's mesenteric border at the points where vasa recta penetrate muscle wall, accounting for 70% of bleeding in right colon?

Diverticula

How do you make the diagnosis of diverticulitis?

Avoid barium enema and endoscopy; Diagnose by history and abdominal or pelvic CT

What are four abdominal radiographic findings of diverticulitis?

-Ileus

-Partially obstructed colon

-Air/fluid level

-Free air if perforated

What is the initial therapy for diverticulitis?

-Intravenous fluids

-Nothing by mouth

-Broad spectrum antibiotics

-NG suction

When is surgery indicated in the treatment of diverticulitis?

Abscess; Obstruction; Fistula;
Perforation; Sepsis

Where are diverticulum most likely to be found?

Diverticulum are most commonly seen in the sigmoid colon

Which disorder is characterized by LLQ pain (cramping or steady), change in bowel habits (diarrhea), fever/chills, anorexia, LLQ mass, nausea/vomiting, dysuria?

Diverticulitis

How often does diverticular bleeding recur?

Approximately 15-20% of patients will have a recurrence of diverticular bleeding within 5 years

What disorder is characterized by saccules of GI mucosa covered by serosa, but not including the muscular layer?

Diverticulosis

Where in the colon is a diverticular bleed most likely to occur?

Approximately 70% occur in the right colon

Which syndrome is caused by delivery of hyperosmotic chyme to the small bowel causing massive fluid shifts into the bowel (normally stomach will decrease osmolality of chyme prior to its emptying)?

Dumping syndrome

What are the typical findings in patients with duodenal ulcers?

Peptic ulcer disease; Mean age 20-40 with M>F; Most common type of PUD; Majority within 2 cm of pylorus; Pathology secondary to increased gastric acid

What disorder is characterized by epigastric pain occurring 3-4 hours after eating, described as burning, aching, boring, gnawing, pressure that awakes the patient from sleep and is relieved by antacids and food?

Duodenal ulcer

Where do duodenal ulcers occur?

90-95% occur in the first portion of the duodenum

What are the gastrointestinal manifestations of systemic sclerosis?

Over 80% of patients with systemic sclerosis have esophageal dysfunction characterized by absent or reduced peristalsis resulting in progressive dysphagia to liquids and solids

What is diffuse esophageal spasm?

Diffuse esophageal spasm is a
neurologic condition in which
peristalsis is significantly impaired by
non-propulsive contractions of the
esophagus resulting in dysphagia of
both liquids and solids

What is one indication that a patient with dysphagia has a neuromuscular mechanism of disease?

Patients with structural abnormalities such as a stricture or tumor present with dysphagia of solids first with progression to liquids. Patients with neuromuscular disorders will often present with onset of concurrent dysphagia to both liquids and solids

What are 5 factors which predispose to worsening encephalopathy in end stage liver disease?

Excessive intestinal nitrogen (GI bleeding); Decreased intestinal motility; Alkalosis; Portal hypertension; Renal failure

What is the diagnosis associated with a corkscrew noted on a barium swallow?

Diffuse esophageal spasm

Familial polyposis coli is characterized by a colon that becomes covered with polyps by the second or third decade of life. The risk of cancer is 100% unless the colon is removed. What is the genetic marker for this disease?

Deletion of APC gene on chromosome 5

What is the inheritance of familial adenomatous polyposis (FAP)?

FAP is inherited autosomal dominant

What are the characteristics of Familial polyposis coli?

This is an autosomal dominant syndrome characterized by production of hundreds of adenomatous polyps within the rectum and colon with onset at puberty with evolution into cancer by age 40-50

Fetor hepaticus is an abnormal musty sweet odor of the breath associated with liver disease. What causes fetor hepaticus?

Abnormal methionine metabolism

What is the most common symptom
of fulminant hepatitis?

Hepatic encephalopathy

What is the disorder characterized by hepatic failure with stage III or IV encephalopathy (deep somnolence or coma) which develops in less than eight weeks in a patient without preexisting liver disease?

Fulminant hepatitis

What is the pathogenesis of
hypoglycemia in the setting of
fulminant hepatic failure?

Decreased gluconeogenesis

What is the most common type of gall stone?

Approximately 75% of gall stones will be cholesterol stones and 25% will be pigment stones

Which disorder is characterized by abdominal distention, vomiting, hypovolemia, and RUQ pain? (40% will show air in the biliary tract)?

Gall stone ileus

Which variant of familial polyposis coli is associated with desmoid tumors, osteomas of skull or mandible, and sebaceous cysts?

Gardner's syndrome (colonic polyposis, bone tumors, soft tissue tumors)

What is the most common cause of
gastric outlet obstruction?

Peptic ulcer disease

What quantity of gastric fluid is normally secreted daily?

The 24 hour secretion of gastric fluid is approximately 2 liters / 24 hours

What is the most common symptom

of intestinal giardiasis?

Abdominal bloating

What is the sensitivity of three stool samples in the workup of possible giardiasis?

Testing three stool samples for ovum and parasites will have about a 90% sensitivity when attempting to make the diagnosis of giardia

Where are gastric ulcers most commonly located?

95% of gastric ulcers are in lesser curvature of the stomach

What are the symptoms of a gastric ulcer?

This disorder is often characterized by abdominal pain that is transiently relieved by foods and antacids.

What is the triad seen with gastric volvulus?

Bouchards triad (emesis, epigastric pain, and inability to pass NG tube)

List 7 causes of lower gastrointestinal bleeding?

Lower gastrointestinal bleeding can be caused by hemorrhoids, anal fissure, diverticulosis, ischemic bowel disease, Meckel's diverticulum (patent omphalomesenteric duct), solitary colonic ulcer, and intussusception

List 8 causes of upper GI bleeding?

Duodenal ulcer; Gastric ulcer;
Anastomotic ulcer; Esophagitis;
Gastritis; Mallory-Weiss tear;
Esophageal varices; Hematobilia

What are the three steps of evaluating acute gastrointestinal hemorrhage?

Determine if the bleed is proximal or distal to ligament of treitz; obtain a plain film of abdomen to rule out obstruction; Perform endoscopy to identify bleeding (esophagogastroduodenoscopy (EGD), sigmoidoscopy)

What is the classic triad of hemobilia?

RUQ pain; Upper GI bleeding;

Jaundice

How is the diagnosis of acute

hepatitis A made?

HAV-IgM

How is the diagnosis of acute hepatitis C made?

The first laboratory finding after infection with Hepatitis C is HCV RNA in the peripheral blood. This typically is found in the peripheral blood within 1-2 weeks of infection.

What are the two diagnostic tests for acute hepatitis B?

HBsAg (hepatitis B surface antigen;
Anti HBc-IgM

What is the first marker for acute

hepatitis B to show in the serum?

First - Hepatitis B surface antigen

What is the incubation period for
Hepatitis A?

The incubation period for Hepatitis A
is 15-45 days

What is the incubation period for Hepatitis B?

The incubation period for Hepatitis B is 30-180 days

What is the term for an infection
with hepatitis D that occurs
simultaneously with hepatitis B?

Coinfection

What percentage of people with hepatitis C develop anti-HCV?

At 6 weeks approximately 70% of patients with hepatitis C infection will have anti HCV.

Does hepatitis A cause cirrhosis or chronic hepatitis?

No

How are hepatitis A IgG antibodies interpreted?

IgG anti hepatitis A antibodies are indicative of an infection with hepatitis A within the preceding months

How are hepatitis A IgM antibodies interpreted?

IgM anti hepatitis A antibodies are indicative of a recent infection with hepatitis A

How long does it take for an acute illness from hepatitis A to resolve?

Acute illness from hepatitis A generally resolves in a period of 2-6 weeks

How often does hepatitis A cause
fulminant hepatitis?

Approximately 1% of patients

Are people with the anti-HBs
antibody protected from infection
with hepatitis B?

Yes, the presence of the anti-HBs is a
marker of immunity from hepatitis B

Does the presence of HBe antigen indicate that the patient is infectious?

Yes, the presence of the HBe antigen indicates that the patient is infectious

How long is the HBe antigen generally seen in the blood of infected patients?

The HBe antigen is generally detectable for 2-6 weeks

How often will HBeAg positive mothers infect their newborns if no intervention is taken?

Approximately 90% will infect their newborns with hepatitis B if no intervention is taken

What does the presence of HBe antigen indicate?

The HBe antigen in the blood indicates that hepatitis B is actively replicating

What is indicated by a positive HBsAg?

The presence of HBsAg indicates an acute or chronic infection with hepatitis B

What is indicated by the presence of
anti-HBc antibody in the serum?

Anti-HBc antibody is an indication of
previous infection with hepatitis B

What is indicated by the presence of anti-HBc?

Anti-HBc is the earliest antibody to develop in the setting of an acute infection

What is indicated by the presence of anti-Hbe?

Anti-Hbe indicates resolution of an acute infection with hepatitis B

When is the HBs-Ag generally detectable after exposure to hepatitis B?

The HBS-Ag generally is detectable at 1-4 months

How long can it take for patients infected with hepatitis C to develop hepatitis C antibodies?

It can take up to a year for some people infected with hepatitis C to develop hepatitis C antibodies

How often will patients with hepatitis C develop chronic hepatitis?

Approximately 80% of patients with hepatitis C will develop chronic hepatitis

What is the most common cause of chronic viral hepatitis?

Hepatitis C

Hemochromatosis is typically treated with phlebotomy. Treated patients will have improvement in splenomegaly, hepatomegaly, liver tests, cardiac function, and skin bronzing. What two symptoms are not improved with phlebotomy?

-Hypogonadism (pituitary infiltration)

-Arthropathy

Describe the pathogenesis of hereditary hemochromatosis?

There is a defect in the ability of intestinal epithelium to block the entry of dietary iron in the presence of excessive iron stores

How often do patients with hemochromatosis have a positive family history?

25% of patients with hemochromatosis have a positive family history

What are the lab findings of hemochromatosis?

The typical lab findings in a patient with hemochromatosis include increased serum iron, increased transfusion saturation >55%, increased serum ferritin, and increased glucose.

What is the best screening test for hemochromatosis?

A transferrin saturation >40% is the best screening test for hemochromatosis

What is the classic triad of hemochromatosis?

Micronodular pigment cirrhosis; Diabetes; Skin pigmentation

Describe first, second, third, and fourth degree hemorrhoids?

First--Do not prolapsed; Second-- Prolapse with defecation and return on their own; Third--Prolapse with defecation or any type of Valsalva and don't return on their own; Fourth-- Cannot be reduced

List six treatments for hemorrhoids

High fiber diet; Anal Hygiene;
Topical steroids; Sitz baths; Rubber
band ligation; Surgical resection

List three common causes of hemorrhoids?

-Constipation/straining

-Portal hypertension

-Pregnancy

Which stage of hepatic encephalopathy is associated with apathy, restlessness, reversal of sleep rhythm, slowed intellect, impaired computational ability, and impaired handwriting?

Stage one hepatic encephalopathy

Which stage of hepatic encephalopathy is characterized by stupor, hyper-reflexia, and extensor plantar responses?

Stage III hepatic encephalopathy

Which stage of hepatic
encephalopathy is associated with
coma (responds only to painful
stimuli)?

Stage IV hepatic encephalopathy

What are two drugs which can

produce hepatic granulomas?

Allopurinol and Sulfonamides

What are four primary benign liver tumors?

Hemangioma; Hepatocellular adenoma (birth control pills and steroids); Focal nodular hyperplasia; infantile hemangioendothelioma

How is blood supplied to the liver?

Arterial --Celiac trunk ---Common hepatic artery

Venous-- Splenic vein ---Superior mesenteric vein ---Portal vein

What is the most common benign liver tumor?

Hepatic hemangioma (do not biopsy)

What is the most common malignant liver tumor?

Metastatic lesions from other primary cancer

Which benign liver tumor is seen in women on birth control pills?

Hepatocellular adenoma

Describe chronic active hepatitis?

This disorder often results in liver failure and/or cirrhosis. Etiology varies. HBV causes minority of cases with or without HDV coinfection, but HAV is not responsible at all. HCV causes majority of cases, drugs occasionally responsible

List five drugs which can cause acute hepatitis?

Acetaminophen; Isoniazid;
Halothane; Chlorpromazine;
Erythromycin

List two metabolic liver diseases that can cause chronic hepatitis?

-Wilson's disease

-Alpha-1 antitrypsin deficiency

The only way to differentiate between chronic active hepatitis and chronic persistent hepatitis is by biopsy. Both diseases can be associated with hepatitis B. Describe the pathology of chronic active hepatitis on biopsy?

Chronic active hepatitis will have piecemeal necrosis, hepatocellular regeneration, and extension of inflammation into the liver lobule.

What are 4 common causes of acute hepatitis?

-Viral (hepatitis A, hepatitis B, hepatitis C, hepatitis D, EBV, CMV)

-Alcohol

-Toxins (CCL4)

-Drugs (Acetaminophen, Isoniazid, Halothane)

What are the common hepatic enzyme levels among viral, toxic, and ischemic hepatitis?

In all of the above the ALT and AST are generally greater than 500

What benign disorder usually follows typical acute hepatitis but may be detected de novo and is characterized by a persistent increase in aminotransferase with vague or no other symptoms, unremarkable LFT's, and rare jaundice?

Chronic persistent hepatitis

Which type of viral hepatitis has 42 nm DNA, a 40-180 day incubation (mean 75), a 33% rate of jaundice, and a 5-10% chronicity rate?

Hepatitis B

What is the pathogenesis and management of hyponatremia secondary to fulminant hepatic failure?

Pathogenesis is related to impaired free water clearance. Management involves monitoring blood electrolyte and fluid balance, and free water restriction

Which area of the intestinal wall has absence of intramural ganglionic cells in Hirschprung's disease?

Meissner's plexus (submucosal);
Auerbach's plexus (myenteric)

Where the haustra and what are their appearance on an abdominal radiograph?

The haustra are found in the colon, and they are not fully circumferential on an abdominal radiograph. This helps to differentiate the colon from the small bowel where the plicae circularis are circumferential

List seven extra intestinal manifestations of inflammatory bowel disease?

Aphthous ulcers; Iritis; Pyoderma granulosa; Erythema nodosum; Clubbing of fingers; Sclerosing cholangitis; Arthritis

Name two conditions that may improve after colectomy in patients with inflammatory bowel disease?

Chronic active hepatitis;
Granulomatous hepatitis

What are 3 medical treatments for inflammatory bowel disease?

Sulfasalazine

Prednisone/steroids

Flagyl for flare ups

What are five indications for surgery in patient with ulcerative colitis?

Toxic megacolon; Cancer prophylaxis; Refractory to treatment; Increased bleeding; Failure of child to grow properly

What are the five factors associated
with fatal outcome of patients with
first attack of ulcerative colitis?

Age >60; Pancolitis; Toxic megacolon;
Hypovolemia; Hypokalemia

What condition is associated with
diarrhea, arthritis, iritis, uveitis, and
erythema nodosum?

Inflammatory bowel disease

What is the colon cancer risk for patients with ulcerative colitis?

2% per year after first ten years of disease

Which inflammatory bowel
disease has discontinuous
involvement?

Crohn's disease

Which inflammatory bowel disease
involves rectum and spreads
proximally in continuous rate without
skip lesions?

Ulcerative colitis

Which inflammatory bowel disease is

associated with anal fistulas?

Crohn's disease

Which inflammatory bowel disease is associated with colonic perforation, toxic megacolon, and cancer?

Ulcerative colitis

Which inflammatory bowel disease is associated with perirectal abscesses, fissures, and fistulas?

Crohn's disease

Which inflammatory bowel disease is associated with skip lesions and is sometimes known as regional enterocolitis?

Crohn's disease

Which inflammatory bowel disease is
confined to the mucosa/submucosa?

Ulcerative colitis

Which inflammatory bowel disease will manifest with deep fissures and fistulas?

Crohn's disease

How is increased psychological stress associated with worsening of irritable bowel syndrome (IBS)?

Psychological stress has been associated with increased intracolonic pressure in normal subjects as well as in IBS. This is thought to lead to increased visceral perception followed by increased intestinal motility.

List 6 symptoms common in irritable bowel syndrome?

Chronic intermittent symptoms;

Intermittent pain, usually LLQ;

Alternating hard stools and diarrhea;

Feeling of incomplete evacuation;

Relief of pain with flatus and bowel

movements

List two factors that are not associated
with irritable bowel syndrome (IBS)
and would help in ruling out IBS?

IBS is not associated with blood in
the stool; IBS will not wake patients
from sleep with pain

What are the 2 pathophysiologic
abnormalities seen in irritable bowel
syndrome?

Increased visceral perception

Altered intestinal motility

What are the laboratory, microbiologic, and histologic markers for irritable bowel syndrome?

There are none

What is the initial workup of irritable bowel syndrome?

History; Physical; Stool analysis; Routine laboratory tests; Proctosigmoidoscopy and/or barium enema to rule out organic disease of colon

What is the most common disease seen by GI specialists?

Irritable bowel syndrome represents approximately half of outpatient visits to gastroenterologists in the United States

Which three symptoms help differentiate irritable bowel syndrome from other gastrointestinal disorders?

Visible abdominal distention; Relief of pain with bowel movements; Looser and more frequent stools with pain

What is seen on colonoscopy in patients with ischemic colitis?

These patients will have findings of friable, edematous, and hemorrhagic colonic mucosa on colonoscopy

What are the typical physical exam
findings of ischemic colitis?

Patients have left lower quadrant
tenderness and rectal bleeding

What are the typical symptoms of ischemic colitis?

Patients generally develop cramping abdominal pain, nausea, diarrhea, and bloody stool

Which two colonic segments are most commonly involved in ischemic colitis?

The most commonly involved segments of colon are the splenic flexure and the rectosigmoid colon

List eight causes of hepatic jaundice?

Drugs; Hypotension; Hypoxia; Hepatitis; Sympathetic inflammation secondary to RLL pneumonia or infarction; Cirrhosis; Right sided heart failure

What are the three mechanisms of predominantly unconjugated hyperbilirubinemia?

Overproduction (hemolysis, ineffective erythropoiesis); Decreased hepatic uptake (Gilbert's disease, drugs (rifampin, contrast dye), neonatal jaundice); Decreased conjugation (Gilbert's disease, Crigler Najjar)

What is the daily secretions of bile?

The 24 hour secretion of bile is
approximately 1 liter

What six mechanisms can cause post hepatic jaundice?

Obstruction (stone); Cholangitis; Cholecystitis; Biliary duct injury; Pancreatitis; Sclerosing cholangitis

Describe the findings of a 72 hour fecal fat analysis on a patient who has fat malabsorption?

Fecal fat greater than 6 g/day on a 72 hour fecal fat analysis is consistent with fat malabsorption

How does small bowel bacterial overgrowth result in fat malabsorption?

Bacterial enzymes deconjugate intraluminal bile salts to free bile acids which are unable to solubilize monoglycerides and free fatty acids into micelles for absorption

What are the common causes of malabsorption?

Malabsorption is commonly related to inadequate digestion, inadequate absorption, lymphatic obstruction, multifactorial, and drug-induced mechanisms

What are the two basic mechanisms of fat absorption?

Pancreatic lipase is activated at a pH 6-8 is responsible for triglyceride hydrolysis in the duodenum producing fatty acids; Bile salts solubilize the fatty acids created by the pancreatic lipase

Where is calcium, folic acid, and
vitamin B12 absorbed?

Proximal small bowel

Which fat soluble vitamins will have impaired absorption when there is impaired fat absorption, such as in bacterial overgrowth or pancreatic lipase insufficiency?

Impaired fat absorption can lead to deficiencies of fat soluble vitamins (Vitamins A, D, E, and K)

What are the treatment options for a Mallory-Weiss tear?

Room temperature water lavage (90% stop bleeding); Electrocautery; Arterial embolization; Surgery

What are three risk factors for development of a Mallory-Weiss tear?

Retching; Alcoholism; Hiatal hernia

What are the three complications of Meckel's diverticula?

Internal hemorrhage (painless) (accounts for 50% of lower GI bleeds in patients < 2 years old); Intestinal obstruction (25%) (Most common complication in adults); Inflammation (perforation possible)

What is the location of a Meckel's diverticula?

Meckel's diverticula are located within two feet of the ileocecal valve on the antimesenteric border of the bowel

What is the most common age of onset of Meckel's diverticula?

The onset is most frequently in first two years of life, but can occur at any age

What is the remnant of omphalomesenteric duct (vitelline duct) which connects the yolk sac to primitive midgut in the embryo?

Meckel's diverticulum

Which disease is characterized by weight loss, post prandial abdominal pain, occult blood, diarrhea, and is commonly associated with digitalis?

Chronic mesenteric ischemia (most commonly secondary to peripheral vascular disease in two or more intestinal arteries)

Which synthetic PGE1 analog decreases gastric acid production and increases mucus and bicarbonate secretion?

Misoprostol (Cytotec)

What is Ogilvie's syndrome?

Acute colonic pseudo-obstruction associated with another medical conditions such as surgery, spinal cord injuries, cardiovascular events, and electrolyte disturbances

Which drug suppresses gastric acid secretion by inhibition H/K ATPase enzyme at the surface of parietal cells?

Omeprazole

Which disorder is characterized by failure of the two pancreatic ducts to fuse, causing the normally small duct of Santorini to act as the main duct?

Pancreatic divisum

List three manifestations of pancreatic and small bowel disease associated with malabsorption?

Night blindness -- Vitamin A deficiency; Ecchymosis -- Vitamin K deficiency; Tetany -- Vitamin D deficiency with secondary hypocalcemia

What is an encapsulated collection of pancreatic fluid with no epithelial cell lining?

Pancreatic pseudocyst

What are the symptoms of a pancreatic pseudocyst?

Epigastric pain, fever, weight loss, palpable epigastric mass, tender epigastrium.

What is the treatment of a pancreatic
pseudocyst?

Treat the pancreatitis. Drain the
pseudocyst after it matures

Which condition is characterized by the decompression of a pseudocyst or abscess into an adjacent organ?

Pancreatic enteric fistula

How long does it take for serum amylase to begin rising after someone develops acute pancreatitis?

The serum amylase will begin to rise in 2-6 hours

How long does the serum amylase remain elevated in patients with acute pancreatitis?

The serum amylase will remain elevated 2-4 days

How long will the serum lipase remain elevated in patients with acute pancreatitis?

The serum lipase will remain elevated for 7-14 days

If the small bowel doesn't produce amylase, why is small bowel injury associated with increases in serum amylase?

Small bowel injury can result in increased permeability of the small bowel mucosa where amylase produced in the pancreas is tightly bound

Is it true that morphine is contraindicated in the treatment of acute pancreatitis because of sphincter of Oddi spasm?

No, there are no clinical studies or evidence to indicate morphine is contraindicated for use in acute pancreatitis. (Am J Gastroenterol 2001 Apr;96(4):1266-72)

List 2 medications associated with acute pancreatitis?

Furosemide (Lasix); Sulfonamides

List seven potential complications of chronic pancreatitis?

Pseudocyst formation; Pancreatic ascites; Common bile duct obstruction; Diabetes mellitus; Splenic vein thrombosis; Exocrine insufficiency; Peptic ulcer

What is the daily secretions of pancreatic fluid?

These secretions are approximately

600 ml / 24 hours

What is the ecchymotic discoloration around the flanks associated with hemorrhagic pancreatitis?

Grey Turner's sign

What is the ecchymotic
discoloration around the
umbilicus associated with
hemorrhagic pancreatitis?

Cullen's sign.

What is the exocrine function of the pancreas?

Secretion of amylase, lipase, trypsin/chymotrypsin, and carboxypeptidase

What is the term for bleeding into parenchyma and surrounding retroperitoneal structures with extensive pancreatic necrosis?

Hemorrhagic pancreatitis (Cullen's - periumbilical bruising, Grey-Turner's -flank bruising)

What tissues are known to be
involved in amylase production other
than the pancreas and salivary
glands?

Tonsils, fallopian tubes, lung, thyroid,
and malignancy are all known to
produce amylase

When does the serum amylase reach peak levels in someone with acute pancreatitis?

The serum amylase will reach peak levels at 12-30 hours

When does the serum lipase begin to rise in patients with acute pancreatitis?

The serum lipase will begin rising in 2-4 hours in a patient with acute pancreatitis

When will the serum lipase reach peak levels in patients with acute pancreatitis?

The serum lipase will reach peak levels at 12-30 hours

Will the serum amylase return to normal sooner than the lipase in patients with acute pancreatitis?

No, the lipase will remain elevated 7-14 days, the amylase generally will return to normal in 2-4 days

What are the two functions of acid secretion in the stomach?

Acid activates pepsin, initiating the first stage of protein digestion; Antibacterial barrier

Can a blood test be used to help diagnose helicobacter pylori infection?

Helicobacter pylori infection in the stomach should result in elevations of IgG and IgA antibodies to helicobacter pylori in the blood

How long does it take for the IgG antibodies to helicobacter pylori to return to normal after adequate treatment for helicobacter pylori testing?

IgG antibodies should decrease by 50% when compared to pretreatment levels within 6 months of treatment

What are the typical findings in a patient presenting with a perforated peptic ulcer?

Patients with perforated peptic ulcers present with acute onset upper abdominal pain, decreased bowel sounds, tympanic sounds over the liver (air), abdominal tenderness, leukocytosis, and free air under the diaphragm on abdominal radiograph.

What is the most common location for a duodenal ulcer?

Approximately 95% of duodenal ulcers are found in the first portion of the duodenum

What is the pathogenesis of gastric ulcer disease?

Normal or decreased gastric acid; Gastric ulcers develop because of a change in mucosal resistance to acid

What is the sensitivity of helicobacter pylori IgG and IgA antibodies in the serum?

Approximately 90%

What type of peptic ulcer disease is characterized by increased acid with increased number of parietal cells, increased responsiveness of the parietal cells to stimulation (food, gastrin, histamine), and increased vagal activity?

Duodenal ulcer disease

Which peptic ulcer disease is seen in the elderly population, not associated with increased acid, often associated with achlorhydria and hypochlorhydria, and must be followed until completely healed?

Gastric ulcer disease

Which peptic ulcer disease peaks in young adults, is associated with helicobacter pylori, excessive acid secretion, and frequent recurrences?

Duodenal ulcer disease

What disorder is characterized by a chronic cholestatic syndrome of unknown etiology with fibrosing inflammation of intra and extra hepatic bile ducts leading to narrowing and eventual obliteration of bile ducts and development of cirrhosis?

Pericholangitis

What disorder, usually diagnosed
with CT scan or ultrasound of the
abdomen, is characterized by
pancreatic edema that usually resolves
spontaneously?

Phlegmon

Where are the plicae circularis and what are their appearance on an abdominal radiograph?

Plicae circularis are the folds in the small bowel and they are circumferential on the abdominal radiograph. This helps differentiate the small bowel from the large bowel where the haustra are not circumferential

How do you use ascites to differentiate portal hypertension as a cause of ascites?

Calculate the serum-to-ascites albumin gradient (serum albumin concentration minus the ascites albumin concentration). A gradient of >1.1 mg/dL is consistent with portal hypertension.

Portal hypertension is caused by distortion of normal parenchyma by regenerating hepatic nodules. What is the most common physical finding?

Splenomegaly

What are the 2 general mechanisms
by which portal hypertension
develops?

Portal hypertension can be caused by
either increased resistance to flow or
increased portal flow.

What are the two endoscopic procedures used to stop variceal bleeding?

Variceal sclerosis with an injection of ethanolamine oleate or sodium tetradecyl; Band ligation which entails placing a rubber ligature around the varix.

Are patients with primary biliary cirrhosis more likely to be female?

Yes, approximately 95% of patients with primary biliary cirrhosis are female

How often do patients with primary
biliary cirrhosis have positive
antimitochondrial antibodies?

Approximately 95% of patients with
primary biliary cirrhosis have
antimitochondrial antibodies

What are the laboratory abnormalities associated with primary biliary cirrhosis?

Primary biliary cirrhosis can cause jaundice secondary to increased conjugated bilirubin. The antimitochondrial antibody is the diagnostic lab finding.

What is the probable diagnosis in a middle aged or elderly female with cirrhosis and history of pruritus, hyperlipoproteinemia, and xanthomas?

Primary biliary cirrhosis

A 43 y/o man has ulcerative colitis, an elevated alkaline phosphatase, and cholestasis. What is one possible unifying diagnosis?

Primary sclerosing cholangitis

What is the most common underlying disease process in a patient with history of inflammatory bowel disease who presents with cirrhosis?

Primary Sclerosing Cholangitis (chronic cholestatic syndrome of unknown etiology characterized by fibrosing inflammation of intra and extra hepatic bile ducts leading to narrowing and obliteration of bile ducts and development of cirrhosis)

What is the result of
antimitochondrial antibody test in
primary sclerosing cholangitis?

Negative

What is the etiology of
pseudomembranous colitis?

Clostridium difficile

Which rare eye disease can be a complication of pancreatitis? It is characterized by a sudden loss of vision thought secondary to occlusion of the posterior retinal artery by granulocytes?

Purtscher's retinopathy

What are the 5 major Ranson's criteria for acute pancreatitis at time of admission?

Age > 55; WBC > 16,000; Glucose > 200; LDH > 2x normal; SGOT > 2x normal

What are Ranson's major criteria used to predict outcome in patients with pancreatitis during <u>initial 48 hours?</u>

Fall in hematocrit > 10%; Serum calcium < 8 mg/dl; Increase in BUN > 5 mg/dl; Arterial PO2 < 60mmhg; Base deficits > 4 meq/liter; Fluid sequestration > 6 liters

What are the 5 components of Reynolds pentad (seen in suppurative cholangitis)?

Fever; Jaundice; RUQ pain; Mental status changes; Shock/sepsis

Which physical exam finding is characterized when palpation of LLQ results RLQ pain?

Rovsing's sign seen with appendicitis

What is Saint's triad?

Cholelithiasis; Hiatal hernia;

Diverticular disease

What is a Shatzki's ring?

A Schatzki's ring is a congenital 2-4 mm structure at the squamocolumnar junction in the distal esophagus which can result in intermittent dysphagia for solids

What causes fibrous thickening of bile duct wall creating beads on a string appearance on contrast study, and commonly presents with progressive obstruction and often leads to cirrhosis and liver failure?

Sclerosing Cholangitis (the etiology is unknown, but 40% are associated with inflammatory bowel disease)

What is the finding of sentinel loops on an abdominal radiograph?

Sentinel loops describe distension and/or air-fluid levels in bowel near a site of abdominal inflammation

Describe the short bowel syndrome?

Malabsorption and diarrhea resulting from extensive bowel resection resulting in <100cm of small bowel remaining.

What is the differential diagnosis for referred shoulder pain from the abdomen related to diaphragmatic inflammation?

Spleen; Perforated ulcer; Abscess

List seven possible etiologies of a small bowel obstruction?

Abdominal surgery; Peritonitis; Generalized sepsis; Electrolyte imbalances (especially hypokalemia); Retroperitoneal hemorrhage; Spinal fractures; Pelvic fractures

What are four clinical parameters that will lower threshold to operate on a small bowel obstruction?

Increased WBC; Fever; Tachycardia; Peritoneal signs

What are the four most common causes of mechanical small bowel disease in adults?

Adhesions (74%); Hernias (8%); Malignancies of small bowel (8%); inflammatory bowel disease

What is the significance of an air fluid level on an abdominal radiograph?

Seen in obstruction and in ileus on an upright abdominal or chest x-ray. It indicates that intraluminal bowel diameter has increased, allowing for separation of fluid and gas

What is one common cause of splenic vein thrombosis?

Pancreatitis

Under what two conditions should a presumptive diagnosis of spontaneous bacterial peritonitis (SBP) be made in a symptomatic patient?

If ascites has a leukocyte count >1000 cells/ul and/or an absolute neutrophil count > 250 cells/ul

What is the hospital mortality rate of spontaneous bacterial peritonitis?

Approximately 30-40%

What is characteristically seen on pathology on a small bowel biopsy in a patient with sprue?

Flat villi with hyperplastic crypts

What is the definition of steatorrhea?

Stool fat >or = to 9 grams/24 hours

Which drug is a disaccharide with negative charged radicals that adhere to positive charged proteins on the surface of the ulcer crater and forms a protective barrier that shields ulcer from acid and pepsin? It requires an acidic environment.

Sucralfate/Carafate (does not work well with antacids or H2 blockers)

What is the main difference between treatment of sigmoid and cecal volvulus?

Cecal (80% require surgery); Sigmoid (majority undergo endoscopic reduction)

Which type of volvulus composes approximately 1/4 of colonic volvulus occurrence?

Cecal volvulus (idiopathic, poor fixation of R colon, seen in young healthy adults)

Describe the typical findings of gastrointestinal arthritis?

Gastrointestinal arthritis is a disorder that involves large joints such as knees and ankles and occurs with 90% of Whipple's disease, 20% Crohn's disease, 15% post intestinal bypass surgery, and 10% ulcerative colitis

Which intestinal lipodystrophy is seen in men 30-60 characterized by anemia, skin pigmentation, joint symptoms, weight loss, diarrhea, and severe malabsorption. It is diagnosed by lymph nodes biopsies showing PAS positive rod bacilli inside macrophages?

Whipple's disease

Whipple's disease is associated with dilated gut lymphatics, weight loss, diarrhea, malabsorption, arthralgia, and abdominal pain. What is the gram negative actinomycete responsible?

Tropheryma whippelii

What is Wilson's disease?

Wilson's disease is a disease of excessive copper deposition in the tissue related to a deficiency of ceruloplasmin which normally functions in copper transport

Describe the direct reacting (free) copper levels in patients with Wilson's disease?

Even though the total copper level is decreased, the indirect copper level is increased

Describe the levels of indirect reacting copper in the serum of patients with Wilson's disease?

Decreased

How often do patients with Wilson's disease present with abdominal manifestations such as hepatosplenomegaly and ascites?

Approximately 67% of patients

How often do patients with Wilson's disease present with neurologic manifestations?

Approximately 60% of patients

How often to patients with Wilson's

disease have Kayser-Fleischer rings?

Approximately 67% of patients

What are causes of decreased serum copper?

Wilson's disease, diarrhea, malnutrition, malabsorption, and Menke's syndrome are all associated with decreased serum copper

What are some conditions associated with increased copper levels in the serum?

Ingestion of copper sulfate, hemochromatosis, malignancy, infection, thyrotoxicosis, estrogens, pregnancy, and primary biliary cirrhosis have been associated with increased serum copper

What is the probable diagnosis in a
22 y/o with corneal limbus
pigmentation and ceruloplasmin level
of 14 mg/dl?

Wilson's disease

Describe the ceruloplasmin levels in
patients with Wilson's disease?

Decreased

What symptoms are most commonly present in patients with Wilson's disease at the time of diagnosis?

These patients often present with neuropsychiatric problems or liver dysfunction

Which type of hereditary cirrhosis can be associated with neurological disorders?

Wilson's disease (hepatolenticular degeneration)

Why do patients with Wilson's disease have decreased total copper in the serum?

There is decreased total copper because of a decrease in the indirect reacting copper

What is the out pouching of esophageal mucosa and submucosa posteriorly through the cricopharyngeal muscle resulting from discoordination between pharyngeal propulsion and cricopharyngeal relaxation?

Zenker's diverticulum

What is the leading cause of
spontaneous bacterial peritonitis?

E. coli

This concludes Gastroenterology Study Guide:
Fast Focus Study Guide

Search Amazon Kindle books to find other study
guides written by

JT Thomas, MD

Internal Medicine Study Guide

Medical Oncology Study Guide

Multiple Myeloma Study Guide

Differential Diagnosis Study Guide

Rheumatology Study Guide

www.ingramcontent.com/pod-product-compliance
Lightning Source LLC
Chambersburg PA
CBHW051851170526
45168CB00001B/69